Best C
Recip
Cookьоок

Make new and updated recipes.
Impress your dinner guests with secret,
mouthwatering recipes from Chipotle, Olive
Garden, Applebee's and more.

Jaqueline Weber

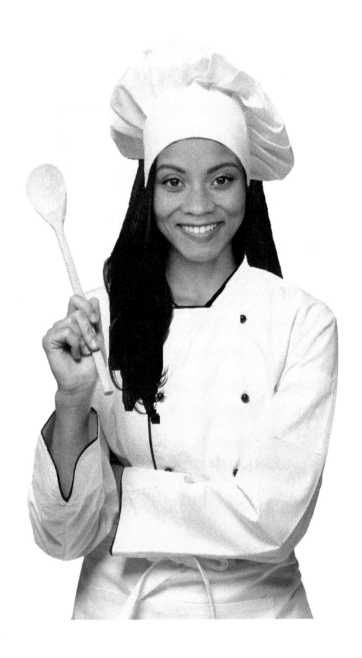

TABLE OF CONTENTS

—
4

INTRODUCTION

One of the most common questions I get is if it's okay to copycat recipes from other people. This is a difficult question to answer because there are several factors that will determine whether or not you can use someone else's recipe.

Copycat recipes have many advantages over original recipes. They are cheaper, they're easier to make, and they taste better. Also, copycat recipes are not copyrighted and therefore you can share them with others for free.

Copycat recipes are a great way to save money and time when cooking at home. The key is to make sure that you are getting the most bang for your buck when it comes to ingredients.

Copycat recipes are a great way for you to get creative with your food and be more adventurous in the kitchen. Making your own recipes can help you save money, and they don't have to be complicated. Copycat recipes are a great way to learn how to cook with ingredients you may not be familiar with. You can get creative and make something unique, or you can follow a recipe and make the dish exactly as it's written. Copycat recipes are a great way to save money and their benefits are numerous.

Copycat recipes are a great way to save money and still get the results you're looking for. This recipe is copied from Reddit, and it's been a hit ever since.

Copycat recipes are great for people that want to try something new but don't have the time or energy to make something from scratch. The recipes in this book are simple and can be made in less than 30 minutes. Copycat Recipes benefits your business by giving you the opportunity to make money. When you're starting out, or even if you're an established company, you can use copycat recipes to get your name out there and drive traffic to your website.

Darlene's copycat recipes are an essential part of the 5 Second Cheesecake brand. Not only do they help her make a quick and easy dessert, but they also give her brand instant credibility. One of the biggest advantages of copycat recipes is that they save you time. Almost all of us are busy and some, especially moms and students, have very limited time in a day. Copycat recipes are a great way to save time and money in the kitchen. You can whip up healthy meals for your family in no time with our copycat recipe's roundup. All you need is a little inspiration.

Copycat recipes are the best way to get new consumers interested in your brand. If you have a hit product, it can be easy to keep everyone happy by producing and selling a copycat version. Copycat recipes are a great way to simplify your cooking and save money. If you're a food blogger or cook, it's important to share your recipes with others in order to gain more followers and exposure. Copycat recipes are great for the following reasons (bolded ones are my favorites): Inexpensive and you can make a lot of them. They're easy to make, especially if you already have the ingredients on hand. 3.

Copycat recipes are not plagiarism, instead they are a way to learn how to make delicious meals. These recipes are especially helpful for those who do not have a cookbook and want to make something tasty and healthy. Copycat recipes are a good way to save money and show customers how much you love their favorite foods. Copycat recipes are a great way to save money and make at home beauty products. This saves you time and money by not having to buy products that you can easily make at home. There are also tons of recipes that look absolutely delicious.

ITALIAN RECIPES

Calzones

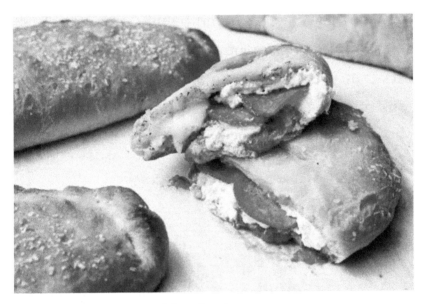

Preparation Time: 10 minutes

Cooking Time: 50 minutes

Servings: 4 calzones

Ingredients:

- 0.75 lb. of pizza dough (either use store bought, or follow the pizza dough recipe in chapter 2 we made for Pizza Pretzels)
- 1 cup of tomato paste

- 1 cup of ricotta cheese
- 1/2 cup of sliced pepperoni
- 1 cup of shredded mozzarella
- 1/2 cup of baby spinach
- Salt to taste
- A pinch of mixed herbs
- All-purpose flour to coat the working surface
- Olive oil for brushing the pastries

Directions:

1. Preheat the oven to 500ºF and lightly grease two baking sheets with cooking spray or oil.

2. Lightly flour a working space and divide the pizza dough into 4 equal quadrants. Roll out one of the dough balls into an 8″ circle. Layer a spoonful of tomato paste into the center of the dough, then add a few spinach leaves, a dollop of ricotta, a few slices of pepperoni, and mozzarella. Season with a pinch of salt and a sprinkle of mixed herbs.

3. Fold the dough over (creating a semicircle), then wet the edges of the semicircle with water and gently press down on the edges with your fingers, to close the filling into the dough. Repeat this process with the other balls of dough.

4. Place the calzones onto the baking trays and brush them with olive oil. Using a knife or scissors, make 3 slits on the top of each of the calzones so that the steam can escape while it's cooking and not get too soggy.

5. Pop the calzones into the oven and bake for 20 minutes. Brush the calzones with oil at the halfway mark. Enjoy it while warm!

Nutrition: Calories 540 Carbohydrates 46.4g Fat 32.8g Protein14.9g

Spaghetti & Meatballs

Preparation Time: 20 minutes

Cooking Time: 1 hour

Servings: 4

Ingredients:

- 1 lb. of spaghetti
- 1 lb. of ground beef (or soya if you're vegetarian)
- 1/3 cup of breadcrumbs
- 1/4 cup of grated parmesan
- 1 egg
- 1 tbsp. of garlic paste
- 1/2 tsp of chili flakes
- 2 tbsps. of olive oil
- 1/2 onion, diced
- 1 can of crushed tomatoes
- 1 bay leaf
- Salt & pepper to taste
- 1/4 cup of chopped parsley
- Extra parmesan and parsley for garnishing

Directions:

1. Fill a large pot ¾ full of water and a pinch of salt. Bring the water to a boil and cook the

spaghetti until it has softened (about 10 minutes).

2. While the spaghetti is cooking, prepare the meatballs. Using a medium-large bowl, mix the beef with the breadcrumbs, parsley, parmesan, egg, garlic, salt, and chili flakes. Mix well and then, using your hands, form about 16 meatballs.

3. Drain the spaghetti once it's softened, using a colander.

4. Bring another medium-large pot to medium heat and drizzle a little bit of oil in it. Place the meatballs into the pot and cook for about 10 minutes, turning them regularly so that they cook evenly. Transfer the meatballs onto a plate.

5. Pour the diced onion into the pot where the meatballs were, and fry for about 5 minutes until the onions have softened. Next, add in the tomatoes and bay leaf, season with salt and pepper, then reduce the heat to a medium low. Add the meatballs back into the pot with the tomato sauce, cover the pot, and leave to simmer for 10 minutes, stirring regularly. Check for the sauce's consistency. If it's thick, it's

ready. If not, leave to simmer for another 5 minutes.

6. Dish the spaghetti onto plates or a serving bowl and top with meatballs and sauce. Sprinkle parmesan on top and garnish with parsley.

7. Bon Appetit!

Nutrition: Calories 738 Carbohydrates86.7g Fat 18.4g Protein 55g

MAIN RECIPES

P.F. Chang's Beef and Broccoli

Preparation Time: 45 minutes

Cooking Time: 15 minutes

Servings: 4

Ingredients

Marinade:

- 1/3 cup oyster sauce
- 2 teaspoons toasted sesame oil
- 1/3 cup sherry
- 1 teaspoon soy sauce
- 1 teaspoon white sugar
- 1 teaspoon corn starch

Beef and Broccoli:

- ¾ pound beef round steak
- 3 tablespoons vegetable oil
- 1 thin slice of fresh ginger root
- 1 clove garlic, peeled and smashed
- 1-pound broccoli, cut into florets

Directions:

1. Incorporate marinade ingredients in a bowl until they have dissolved. Marinate the beef in the mixture for 30 minutes. Sauté the ginger and garlic in hot oil for a minute. When the oil is flavored, remove the garlic and ginger and add in the broccoli. Continue cooking the broccoli until tender.

2. Once cooked, situate it to a bowl and set aside. Pour the beef and the marinade into the pan in which you cooked the broccoli and continue cooking until beef is cooked, or about 5 minutes. Pour the broccoli back in and keep cooking for another 3 minutes. Serve.

Nutrition: 331 Calories 21.1g Total Fat 21.7g Protein

Outback's Secret Seasoning Mix for Steaks

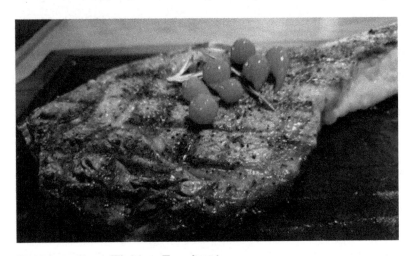

Preparation Time: 5 minutes

Cooking Time: 10 minutes

Servings: 3

Ingredients

Seasoning:

- 4–6 teaspoons salt
- 4 teaspoons paprika
- 2 teaspoons ground black pepper
- 1 teaspoon onion powder
- 1 teaspoon garlic powder
- 1 teaspoon cayenne pepper
- ½ teaspoon coriander

- ½ teaspoon turmeric

Directions:

1. Blend all the seasoning ingredients in a bowl. Rub the spice blend into the meat on all sides and let rest for 15-20 minutes before cooking.

Nutrition: 16.4 Calories 0.5g Total Fat 3.5g Carbohydrates

Taco Bell's Chalupa

Preparation Time: 40 minutes

Cooking Time: 10 minutes

Servings: 8

Ingredients

Tortillas:

- 2½ cups flour
- 1 tablespoon baking powder
- ½ teaspoon salt
- 1 tablespoon vegetable shortening
- 1 cup milk
- Oil, for deep frying

Filling:

- 1 tablespoon dried onion flakes
- ½ cup water
- 1-pound ground beef
- ¼ cup flour
- 1 tablespoon chili powder
- 1 teaspoon paprika
- 1 teaspoon salt
- Some oil for frying

For Garnishing:

- Some sour cream
- Some lettuce, shredded

- Some cheddar cheese or Monterey Jack cheese
- Some tomato, diced

Directions:

2. Combine the flour, baking powder, and salt. Stir in the vegetable shortening and mix. Then add the milk and continue mixing. Portion the dough into 8 parts, and then shape them into 8 6-inch tortillas.

3. Deep fry the tortillas until golden brown. Set aside to cool. Start making the filling. Place the onion flakes in the water and set aside for 5 minutes. Mix the rest of the filling ingredients (except the oil) together until combined. Add in the onion with the water and continue mixing. Heat the oil in a skillet, and then cook the entire beef mixture until the beef browns.

4. Now, assemble your Chalupas. In the tortillas, place the following by layers:

5. Cooked beef mixture; Sour cream; Lettuce; Cheese; and lastly Tomatoes.

6. Serve on a plate.

Nutrition: 424.9 Calories 15.8g Total Fat 21.6g Protein

Chili's Baby Back Ribs

Preparation Time: 15 minutes

Cooking Time: 3 hours 30 minutes

Servings: 4

Ingredients

Pork:

- 4 racks baby-back pork ribs

Sauce:

- 1½ cups water
- 1 cup white vinegar
- ½ cup tomato paste
- 1 tablespoon yellow mustard
- 2/3 cup dark brown sugar packed
- 1 teaspoon hickory flavored liquid smoke
- 1½ teaspoons salt
- ½ teaspoon onion powder
- ¼ teaspoon garlic powder
- ¼ teaspoon paprika

Directions:

1. Combine all of the sauce ingredients and then bring to a boil. Let it simmer for 45 to 60 minutes, stir it occasionally. When it's done, preheat oven at 300 degrees. Cover the 1 rack of ribs with aluminum foil. Put the ribs on top.

2. Take out the sauce from heat and start glazing over the ribs.

3. When it is completely covered, and transfer it on the baking pan with the foil opening facing upwards. Do it again for the remaining racks and bake it for 2½ hours. When it is almost done, prepare your grill at medium heat then cook both sides. Brush some more sauce on each side and grill for another minutes. Don't overcook. Once done, serve with extra sauce.

Nutrition: 645 Calories 43.8g Total Fat 51.5g Protein

Applebee's Honey Barbecue Sauce with Riblets

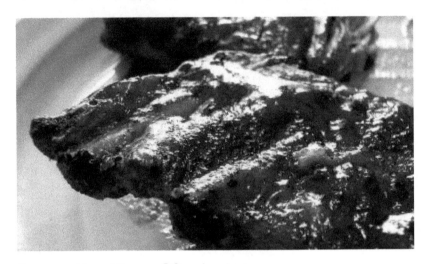

Preparation Time: 20 minutes

Cooking Time: 3 hours 30 minutes

Serving: 4

Ingredients

Honey Barbecue Sauce:

- 1 cup ketchup
- ½ cup corn syrup
- ½ cup honey
- ¼ cup apple cider vinegar
- ¼ cup water
- 2 tablespoons molasses
- 2 teaspoons dry mustard
- 2 teaspoons garlic powder

- 1 teaspoon chili powder
- 1 teaspoon onion powder

Meat:

- 2¼ pounds pork Riblets
- Salt
- Pepper
- Garlic
- ¼ teaspoon liquid smoke flavoring
- 1 teaspoon water

Directions:

1. Season the riblets with the salt, garlic, and pepper based on your preferences, then sear them on a grill until the meat starts to separate from the bone. While doing this, preheat the oven to 275F. Mix the water and liquid smoke flavoring into a deep pan and place the ribs on an elevated rack inside—make sure that the liquid does not touch the ribs.

2. Seal with two layers of foil and bake for 2 to 5 hours and the number of riblets you have. Internal temperature of the meat must be at 155 degree all throughout.

3. While waiting for the riblets to cook, prepare the sauce by mixing all of the sauce ingredients together and simmering for 20 minutes. When

the sauce is done cooking, transfer to a bowl and set aside. When the ribs are done cooking, sear them on a grill until the marrow starts sizzling. Situate ribs on a plate and cover generously with the sauce.

Nutrition: 1110 Calories 57g Total Fat 63g Protein

Cracker Barrel's Green Beans with Bacon

Preparation Time: 10 minutes

Cooking Time: 45 minutes

Servings: 6

Ingredients

- ¼ pound sliced bacon, cut into 1-inch pieces
- 3 cans (14.5 ounces each) green beans, with liquid
- ¼ yellow onion, peeled, chopped
- 1 teaspoon granulated sugar
- ½ teaspoon salt
- ½ teaspoon fresh ground black pepper

Directions:

1. Half-cook the bacon in a saucepan—make sure it does not get crispy. Add the green beans with the liquid to the browned bacon and season with salt, pepper, and sugar. Top the green beans with the onion and then cover the pan until the mixture boils. Decrease the heat and let mixture to simmer for another 45 minutes before serving.

Nutrition: 155.3 Calories 9g Total Fat 6g Protein

Café Rio's Pork

Preparation Time: 10 minutes

Cooking Time: 9 hours

Servings: 10

Ingredients

For the Marinade:

- 3 pounds boneless pork loin
- 12 ounces Coca Cola
- ¼ cup brown sugar

For the Seasoning:

- 1 teaspoon garlic salt
- 1 teaspoon onion salt
- 1 teaspoon chili powder
- 1 teaspoon cumin, ground
- 12 ounces Coca Cola

For the Sauce:

- 12 ounces Coca Cola
- ¾ cup brown sugar
- ½ teaspoon chili powder
- ½ teaspoon ground cumin
- 1 can (4 ounces) green chili, ground
- 1 can (10 ounces) red enchilada sauce

Directions:

2. Mix the Coca Cola and sugar in an airtight container or sealable plastic bag to make the marinade.
3. Massage the marinade into the pork. Situate it in the container to marinate for at least 8 hours.
4. Place the pork into a slow cooker and cover with all of the seasoning ingredients in the order specified. Cook the pork at low for 8 hours.
5. After cooking, shred the pork and remove the liquid from the slow cooker. Put the shredded pork to the slow cooker again. Place all of the sauce ingredients in a food processor or blender. Blend well to create the sauce. Pour the sauce over the pork, and then cook the entire mixture for another 30 minutes. Transfer to a bowl and serve.

Nutrition: 317 Calories 7g Total Fat 28g Protein

Ruth Chris's Filet Mignon with Béarnaise Sauce

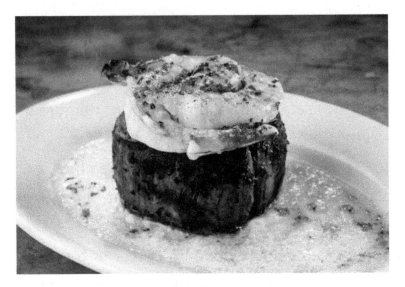

Preparation Time: 10 minutes

Cooking Time: 40 minutes

Servings: 4

Ingredients

Vinegar Reduction:

- 2 tablespoons tarragon vinegar
- 2 teaspoons fresh lemon juice
- 2 teaspoons shallots, finely chopped
- 1 teaspoon dried tarragon
- Fresh ground black pepper, to taste

Sauce:

- 2 large egg yolks

- ¼ cup water
- Salt, to taste
- 2 teaspoons fresh tarragon, chopped
- 2 teaspoons fresh chervil, chopped (optional)
- ½ cup unsalted butter, melted

Steak:

- 4 filet mignon steaks. about 8 ounces each

Directions:

1. Mix all of the vinegar reduction ingredients together and bring to a boil over medium to high heat.
2. When the vinegar mixture starts to boil, lower the heat and allow the mixture to simmer until most of the liquid evaporates. When only small bubbles of liquid are left, remove the vinegar reduction from heat and set aside.
3. Let the water to simmer in the bottom part of a double boiler while whisking the egg yolks and water in the top part. Place the top part over the simmering water, making sure that the water does not touch the bottom of the bowl.
4. Pour the vinegar reduction into the egg mixture and whisk until the entire mixture reaches 284F. Remove the mixture from heat, but continue

whisking. Slowly pour in the melted butter while continuing to whisk the mixture.

5. Add in the remaining sauce ingredients and continue stirring. Set the Béarnaise sauce aside, keeping it warm at 220F. Sprinkle the steaks with salt and pepper while prepping the broiler for 10 minutes. Broil the steaks to your preference. Situate the steaks in a warm plate, pour ¼ cup of Béarnaise sauce, and serve.

Nutrition: 340 Calories 8g Total Fat 201g Protein

P.F. Chang's Spare Ribs

Preparation Time: 5 minutes

Cooking Time: 25 minutes

Servings: 2

Ingredients

Sauce:

- 1 cup ketchup
- 1 cup light corn syrup
- ½ cup hoisin sauce
- ½ cup water
- 1/3 cup light brown sugar, packed
- 2 tablespoons onions, minced
- 1 tablespoon rice vinegar

Ribs:

- 12 to 16 cups water
- 2 teaspoons salt
- 1 rack pork spareribs
- 4 cups vegetable oil
- 1 teaspoon sesame seeds, for garnish
- 1 tablespoon green onion, diced, for garnish

Directions:

1. Stir in all of the sauce ingredients and wait it to boil then let it simmer for 5 minutes. Set aside. Transfer the water and salt into a large pot then

let it boil. In the meantime, clean the spare ribs and take out the excess fat.

2. When it starts to boil, transfer all the ribs into the water and continue boiling for 14 minutes. Drain and set aside. Cook the oil at 375 degrees then put 4 to 6 ribs in it and cook for 6 minutes.

3. Do it again until all the ribs are fried. Combine the fried ribs and the sauce over medium heat. Let it simmer at least a minute. Place the ribs to a plate and serve with rice. Topped the ribs with the sesame seeds and green onions.

Nutrition: 1344 Calories 77.2g Total Fat 52.5g Protein

Boston Market's Meatloaf

Preparation Time: 10 minutes

Cooking Time: 1 hour 25 minutes

Servings: 8

Ingredients

Sauce:

- 1 cup tomato sauce
- 1½ tablespoons barbecue sauce
- 1 tablespoon sugar

Meatloaf:

- 1½ pounds lean ground sirloin
- 6 tablespoons all-purpose flour
- ¾ teaspoon salt
- ½ teaspoon onion powder
- ¼ teaspoon ground black pepper
- 1 dash garlic powder

Directions:

1. Preheat the oven to 400F; and situate ground sirloin in bowl.
2. Incorporate sauce ingredients together then simmer over medium heat. Once simmering, pull away from heat. Keep aside 2 tablespoons of the sauce and pour the rest over the meat. rub the sauce into the meat, marinating it well.

3. Stir in rest of the meatloaf ingredients into the meat mixture then continue kneading until the spices are fully incorporated into the meat. Situate meat into your loaf pan and cover with foil. Bake for 30 minutes.

4. Pull out pan from the oven and drain the fat before cutting the meatloaf into 8 equal portions.

5. Fill in set-aside sauce over the top of the meatloaf and return it to the oven for extra 25 to 30 minutes. Situate meatloaf to a plate and let cool before serving.

Nutrition: 210.1 Calories 10.9g Total Fat 18.3g Protein

SNACK RECIPES

Wendy's Copycat Keto Chili

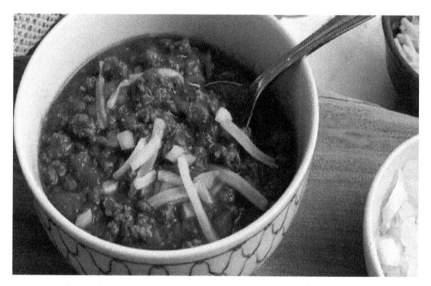

Preparation Time: 27 minutes

Cooking Time: 41 minutes

Servings: 8

Ingredients:

- cups of ground beef
- 2/3 cup of diced celery
- 1/2 cup of diced red capsicum
- 1/2 cup of diced green capsicum

- 1 1/2 cups of diced yellow onion
- 1 cup of chopped tomatoes
- 1 1/2 cups of tomato juice
- 2 cups of mashed tomatoes
- 1 1/2 tsp. of Worcestershire sauce
- 3 tbsp. of chili powder
- 2 tsp. of erythritol, granular
- 1 tsp. sea salt
- 1 tsp. of garlic (powder)
- 1 tsp. of cumin
- 1/2 tsp. of oregano
- 1/2 tsp. of black pepper

Direction

1. Brown the ground beef in a big bowl until it is cooked. Save about two spoonful of fat and drain the remainder of the fat
2. Put the garlic, celery, black bell peppers, and tomatoes into the beef bowl. Cook for another five minutes, over medium-high heat
3. Add tomato juice, the diced tomatoes, the Worcestershire sauce, and all the seasonings. Cover and cook for 1 to 1 1/2 hours, sometimes stirring

Nutrition 225 Calories 10g Protein 12g Fat

PF Chang's Copycat Keto Lettuce Wraps

Preparation Time: 9 minutes

Cooking Time: 13 minutes

Servings: 3

Ingredients:

Lettuce Wraps' ingredients:

- cups of minced turkey
- 1 tbsp. of olive oil
- 2 tsp. of dried minced onion
- 1/4 tsp. of sea salt
- 1/4 tsp. of black pepper
- 3 green onions, thinly sliced
- 1/4 cup of chopped shiitake mushrooms
- 1/2 cup of diced jicama
- Living butter lettuce

Sauce's ingredients:

- 3 tbsp. of soy sauce (less sodium)
- 2 cloves garlic should be minced
- 1/2 tsp. of ginger paste
- 1 tsp. of sesame oil
- 1 tsp. of rice vinegar
- 1 tsp. of brown swerve sweetener

- 1 tsp. of almond butter, natural

Direction

1. Put all ingredients in a small bowl whisk and set aside
2. Heat olive oil in a skillet on the stove. Crumble and cook the minced turkey on medium heat
3. Season with chopped onion, sea salt and black pepper
4. Then add green onion, jicama, and mushrooms
5. Add mushroom with meat until mushroom becomes soft. Mix sauce with meat mixture
6. Add mixture above lettuce pieces and have fun!

Nutrition 188 Calories 26g Proteins 12g Fat

Turkey and Provolone Jimmy John's Unwich

Preparation Time: 8 minutes

Cooking Time: 13 minutes

Servings: 4

Ingredients:

For each Unwich:

- 2 pieces of sliced turkey, ¼ cup
- 1 slice provolone cheese, 1/8 cup
- 3 slices tomato, ¼ cup
- 10 slices of cucumber, ¼ cup
- 1/2 small avocado, 2 cups
- pinch sea salt
- pinch black pepper
- 1 tsp. of real mayonnaise
- 1 tsp. of yellow mustard
- 2-3 large pieces, iceberg lettuce

Direction

1. Place 2-3 leaves of lettuce in a row overlapping each other
2. Start with the meat and cheese, and layer all sandwich ingredients in the middle, but a little

bit closer to lettuce. This tip will make it easier to roll up at the end

3. Tightly wrap up lettuce like a burrito, folding the ends in, so it will be secured. Then tightly wrap in a couple of squares of parchment paper. You may secure with edible tape

4. The easiest way to enjoy is to start at one side and tear the paper down as you eat! Enjoy!

Nutrition 200 Calories 22g Proteins 5g Fat

KFC Low Carb Chicken Pot Pie

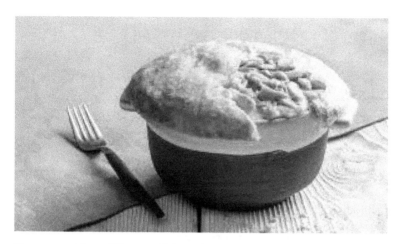

Preparation Time: 20 minutes

Cooking Time: 3 hours

Servings: 8

Ingredients:

Filling:

- 3/4 cup of heavy whipping cream
- 2 tbsp. of butter
- 1/2 cup mixed veggies
- 1/4 of diced small onion
- 1/4 tsp. of pink sea salt
- 1/4 tsp. of black pepper
- 2 garlic cloves minced
- 1 cup of chicken broth
- 1 tsp. of chicken seasoning
- 1/4 tsp. of rosemary

- Pinch thyme
- 2 1/2 cups of diced cooked chicken
- 1/4 tsp. of xanthan gum

Crust:

- 4 eggs
- 4 ½ tsp. of melted and cooled butter
- 2 tbsp. of full fat sour cream
- 1/4 tsp. of sea salt
- 1 cup of cheddar cheese
- 1/3 cup of mozzarella cheese
- 1/4 tsp. of baking powder
- 1/3 cup of coconut flour
- Parsley

Direction

1. Cook all of chicken for 3 hours on maximum in the slow cooker or 6 hours on small
2. Preheat oven to 400 F
3. Sautee garlic cloves, onion, mixed vegetables, sea salt, and black pepper in 2 tbsp. of butter in a heavy skillet for 5 minutes or until translucent onions
4. Stir in thick whipping cream, chicken stock, seasoning meat, thyme, and rosemary
5. Add the xanthan gum on top and boil for 5 minutes to thicken the sauce. Be sure to cover

the broil because else the liquid would evaporate. With this dish, you will need a ton of moisture, or it will be dry!

6. Add grilled chicken
7. Combine melted butter, eggs, sea salt, and sour cream in a bowl to produce the breading
8. Add the mixture with the coconut flour and baking powder, and stir until combined
9. Stir in the cheese
10. Drop flour into the chicken pot pie by dollops. Must not stretch it out as if the coconut flour would drain so much of the moisture
11. Bake for 15–20 min in a 400-degree oven
12. Heat the oven to broil and switch to the top shelf chicken pot pie. Broil for 1-2 minutes until well browned on bread topping. Sprinkle over with fresh parsley

Nutrition 297 Calories 12g Proteins 17g Fat

The Greyhound Café's Copycat Mozzarella Chicken

Preparation Time: 9 minutes

Cooking Time: 22 minutes

Servings: 2

Ingredients:

- 2 cups of boneless skinless chicken breasts
- 1 tbsp. of Italian seasoning
- 1 tsp. of paprika
- 1/2 tsp. of onion powder
- Sea salt and black pepper, to taste
- 1 tbsp. of olive oil
- 1 chopped onion
- 4 cloves of minced garlic
- Fire-roasted pepper, one pepper (chopped)
- 2 cups of tomato puree
- 2 tbsp. of tomato paste
- Pinch crushed red chili flakes
- 3/4 cup of shredded mozzarella
- Parsley: to garnish

Direction

1. Arrange the oven shelf down to the bottom. Preheat broiler on medium heat

---

2. Use Italian seasoning (2 tsp.) onion powder, paprika, sea salt and black pepper to season the chicken.
3. Place oil over medium heat in a skillet. Let the chicken cook on both sides until browned and all of it all is cooked through. Transfer to a plate and let it sit
4. Let the onion cook in the same saucepan until it looks clear (about 3-4 minutes) remove any brown bits from the saucepan's bottom, then add the garlic and cook until it is fragrant. Add black pepper (or capsicum) roasted with fire, crushed tomatoes, tomato paste, and crushed red black pepper flakes and remaining Italian seasoning. To blend properly, give it a quick swirl
5. Bring to a boil and allow the sauce to thicken (about 4 minutes) while stirring occasionally
6. Arrange the Chicken in the sauce with 2-3 tbsp. of mozzarella cheese per breast and then finish each breast. Transfer to the oven and broil for 1-2 minutes or browned and bubbling before the cheese
7. Garnish, then top with parsley

Nutrition 309 Calories 37g Proteins 9g Fat

Olive Garden Beef and Chorizo Low Carbohydrate Empanadas

Preparation Time: 7 minutes

Cooking Time: 24 minutes

Servings: 2

Ingredients:

Filling:

- 2 hardboiled eggs chopped
- 1 cup of minced beef
- 1 cup of pork sausage chorizo
- 1/2 cup of diced onion
- 8 green olives, chopped
- 2 cloves of garlic (minced)
- 2 tbsp. of tomato paste
- Sea salt and black pepper according to your taste
- 3 pieces of chopped onions

For Dough

- 1 large egg
- 1 1/2 of cups of shredded mozzarella cheese
- 3 tbsp. of cream cheese
- 3/4 cup of almond flour
- 1 tsp. of garlic (powder)

- 1 tsp. of onion powder
- 1 tsp. of Italian seasoning
- Sea salt: to taste

Direction

1. Add the minced beef, garlic, pork chorizo, onion, sea salt, and black pepper to a large skillet. Stir on medium-high heat until the meat has been cooked completely. Drain extra Fat and combine with a puree of tomatoes. Mix well for another 5 minutes

2. Move the mixture to a pot; add in the eggs, olives, and green onions. Set it aside

For Dough:

1. Combine cream cheese, mozzarella cheese in a big mixing bowl microwave for 1 minute. Stir to mix and add one extra minute to microwave

2. Combine with almond flour, garlic powder, egg, onion powder, and Italian seasoning with black pepper and sea salt. Mix until all the components are combined properly

3. Combining these two

4. With parchment paper, line two rimmed baking sheets. Stretch the dough all over one of the sheets into a thin layer

5. To make circles into the dough using the edge of a bowl. Drop the rings onto the other layer of baking

6. Make the dough into a ball again, and then repeat until you have 12 circles

7. Oven preheat to 425 F

8. Spoon the mixture of meat into the plate. Fold the dough above the meatball and press the sides. Use a fork to press the sides

9. Bake for twelve minutes

Nutrition: 344 Calories26g Protein 25g Fat

Fluffy's Kitchen Low Carb Keto Biscuits

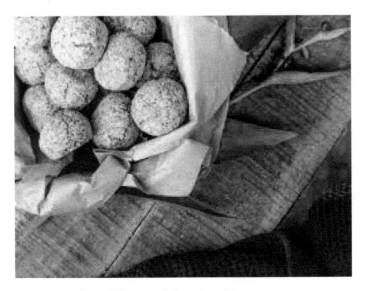

Preparation Time: 12 minutes

Cooking Time: 14 minutes

Servings: 6

Ingredients:

- 2 eggs
- 1 1/2 cups of almond flour
- 2 tsp. of cream of tartar
- 1 tsp. of baking soda
- 1/2 tsp. of sea salt
- 1 cup of shredded mozzarella
- 4 tbsp. of softened butter
- 1/4 cup of heavy whipping cream

Direction

1. Preheat oven to 400 ° F
2. Add together the almond flour, tartar cream, baking soda, and sea salt in a large bowl
3. Using a hand mixer, whisk mozzarella, cheese, eggs, and heavy whipping cream together in a small bowl until well combined
4. Add dry ingredients to the bowl of wet ingredients and start stirring until all ingredients are thoroughly mixed with the hand mixer
5. Spray the muffin sheet with a non-stick cooking mist
6. Dollop dough into separate muffin tin molds, utilizing a greased spoon
7. Bake for 13-15 minutes before the biscuits are golden brown
8. Serve hot, and have fun

Nutrition 157 Calories 8g Proteins 7g Fat

Red Lobster Buffalo Chicken Wings

Preparation Time: 68 minutes

Cooking Time: 55 minutes

Servings: 12

Ingredients:

- 12 pieces of organic chicken wings
- 6 tbsp. of butter
- 1/2 cup of hot sausage (Tapatio)

Direction

1. Bring almost 1 inch of water to a boil in large pot
2. In a steam holder, place all wings and put it into the pan
3. Cover and let it simmer; steam the wings for 10
4. After cooking, place wings on a cooling rack over paper towels and cool in the refrigerator for 1 hour
5. Let the oven hear to 425° F
6. Throw paper towels away and place parchment paper on a cooling rack
7. Bake wings for 20 minutes
8. Flip the wings and bake for another 20 minutes

9. Melt butter in the microwave for 1 minute, meanwhile wings are baking and add to a big bowl. Mix within the hot sauce
10.   After then put the wings into the sauce and keep it covered

Nutrition 140 Calories 22g Proteins 5g Fat

Red Lobster Wild-Caught Snow Crab Legs

Preparation Time: 4 minutes

Cooking Time: 8 minutes

Servings: 4

Ingredients:

- 4 cups of wild-caught snow crab legs
- Lemon slices
- 1cup of water
- 1/3 cup of sea salted grass-fed butter

Direction

1. Put the metal stand under your Instant Pot
2. Then mix 1 cup of water
3. Place the crab legs in the bowl
4. Place the cover onto the Instant Pot and close the lid
5. Click the "Manual," and adjust the duration to three minutes
6. Let the pressure release easily as soon as the Instant Pot starts to beep
7. May use tongs to transfer the legs of cooked crabs to a serving platter
8. Serve with butter and mint!

Nutrition 200 Calories 22g Proteins 8g Fat

KFC Creamy Low-Carb Coleslaw

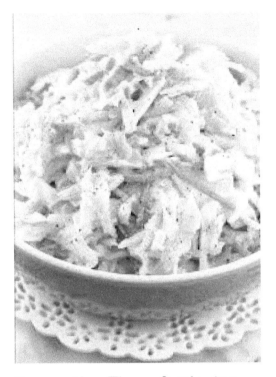

Preparation Time: 9 minutes

Cooking Time: 12 minutes

Servings: 4

Ingredients:

- 2-4 tbsp. of erythritol
- ¼ cup of coleslaw mix
- 1/8 cup of diced onion
- 1 tsp. of garlic powder
- ¼ cup of mayonnaise
- ¼ cup of sour cream

- 1 tbsp. of lemon juice
- 2 tsp. of celery seed
- 2 tbsp. of vinegar
- Sea salt and black pepper

Direction

1. Chop the onion roughly. Add all ingredients to food processor except coleslaw mix and pulse to blend
2. You may pour coleslaw mix to a food processor and mix
3. Cover it and store in the refrigerator
4. It will taste even better!
5. In case of no food processor
6. Finely slice the onion
7. Mix all ingredients but not coleslaw mix and whisk in a small bowl to finely combine chopped coleslaw mix
8. Skip the chopping (optional)
9. Pour the combination of wet ingredients over the coleslaw. Combine. Cover it and store it in the fridge
10.   You can double the recipe for a larger meal to prepare

Nutrition   90   Calories   2g   Proteins   8g   Fat

SAUCE AND DRESSING RECIPES

Kraft Thousand Island Dressing

Preparation Time: 5 minutes

Cooking Time: 0 minute

Servings: 16

Ingredients

- 1 cup mayonnaise
- ¼ cup ketchup
- 2 tablespoons white vinegar
- 4 teaspoons white sugar
- 2 teaspoons sweet pickle relish, minced
- 2 teaspoons white onion, finely chopped or minced
- ¼ teaspoon sea salt
- ¼ teaspoon black pepper

Directions

1. Take a large bowl and combine all the ingredients in it. Mix well. Serve.

Nutrition 67 Calories 4.9g total fat 6g carbohydrates

Newman Own's Creamy Caesar Salad Dressing

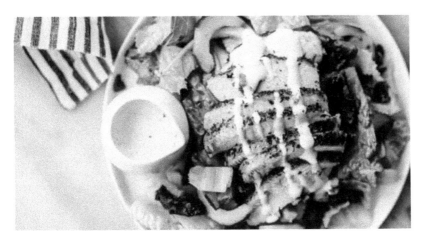

Preparation Time: 5 minutes

Cooking Time: 0 minute

Servings: 10

Ingredients

- 2 cups mayonnaise
- 6 tablespoons white vinegar, distilled
- ¼ cup Parmesan cheese, grated
- 4 teaspoons Worcestershire sauce
- 1 teaspoon lime juice
- 1 teaspoon dry mustard, ground
- 1/3 teaspoon salt, or to taste
- ½ teaspoon garlic powder
- ½ teaspoon onion powder
- ½ teaspoon black pepper, freshly ground

- 1 pinch basil, dried
- 1 pinch oregano, dried

Directions

1. Take an electric mixer and blend all the ingredients until smooth. Chill the prepared dressing for a few hours before severing. Enjoy.

Nutrition 215 Calories 17.4g total fat 2.3g Protein

Bull's Eye Original BBQ Sauce

Preparation Time: 20 minutes

Cooking Time: 15 minutes

Servings: 4

Ingredients

- 1½ cups tomato ketchup
- ½ cup Worcestershire sauce
- 5 tablespoons butter, melted
- ¼ cup white vinegar
- 1 tablespoon yellow mustard
- ¼ cup onions, finely minced
- 2 tablespoons hickory liquid smoke
- ½ teaspoon Tabasco sauce
- 1 cup sugar, brown
- 1 tablespoon white sugar
- Salt, to taste

Directions

1. Incorporate ingredients in a saucepan and heat it over medium heat. Simmer the ingredients for 15 minutes, stirring occasionally. Put off the heat and let the sauce get cold. The sauce is ready.

Nutrition 112 Calories 13.7g total fat 20.5g carbohydrates

Kraft Miracle Whip

Preparation Time: 20 minutes

Cooking Time: 15 minutes

Servings: 2

Ingredients

- 4 egg yolks
- 1/3 teaspoon salt
- 2 tablespoons powdered sugar
- 6 tablespoons lemon juice
- 2 cups oil
- 2 tablespoons cornstarch
- 2 teaspoons dry mustard
- 1 cup boiling water
- ¼ cup vinegar
- Table salt, to taste

Directions

2. Take a blender and add egg yolks along with salt, sugar, and half of lemon juice. Blend for few seconds until combined. While the blender is running, start adding the oil, a few drops at a time.

3. Add the remaining lemon juice. Turn off the blender. In a bowl, mix together cornstarch, water, mustard, and vinegar.

4. Mix until a smooth paste is formed. Pour the bowl ingredients into a pan. Cook on low heat until thickened. Slowly add this cooked mixture into the blender.

5. Turn on the blender and combine all the ingredients well. Transfer to a jar and let cool in the refrigerator.

Nutrition 717 Calories 7.6g total fat 0.6g carbohydrates

Hellman's Mayonnaise

Preparation Time: 15 minutes

Cooking Time: 0 minute

Servings: 2

Ingredients

- 3 large egg yolks
- 1 teaspoon dry mustard
- 1 teaspoon salt
- ½ teaspoon cayenne pepper
- 1½ cups canola oil
- 4–6 tablespoons lemon juice

Directions

1. Add mustard and egg yolks into a blender and pulse until combined. While the blender is blending set the speed to low and start adding the oil very slowly.
2. Stop the blender and scrape down the mayonnaise. Add the lemon juice and remaining oil. Keep on blending until combined. At the end add salt and cayenne pepper. Mix and serve.

Nutrition 362 Calories 39.1g total fat 3.4g Protein

Heinz Ketchup

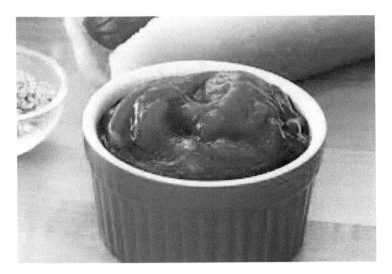

Preparation Time: 25 minutes

Cooking Time: 20 minutes

Servings: 4

Ingredients

- 1 cup tomato paste
- 1/3 cup light corn syrup
- ½ cup white vinegar
- 1/3 cup water
- 2 tablespoons sugar
- Salt, to taste
- 1/3 teaspoon onion powder
- ¼ teaspoon garlic powder

Directions

1. Combine all the ingredients in a saucepan. Put on the heat and let the liquid simmer for 20 minutes. Put off the heat and let the mixture cool down. Store in airtight glass jar or serve with French fries.

Nutrition 78 Calories 0.2g total fat 1.4g Protein

Hidden Valley Original Ranch Dressing

Preparation Time: 10 minutes

Cooking Time: none

Servings: 6

Ingredients

- 1 cup mayonnaise
- 1 cup buttermilk
- 1 teaspoon parsley flakes, dried
- ½ teaspoon black pepper, ground
- 1/3 teaspoon sea salt
- ¼ teaspoon garlic powder
- ¼ teaspoon onion powder
- 2 pinches of thyme, dried

Directions

1. Using a blender, incorporate all the ingredients in it. Pulse until smooth. Transfer to a glass jar and chill in refrigerator before serving.

Nutrition 170 Calories 13.5g total fat 1.8g Protein

Lawry's Taco Seasonings

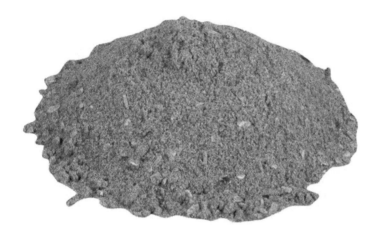

Preparation Time: 10 minutes

Cooking Time: 0 minute

Servings: 2

Ingredients

- 2 tablespoons flour
- 2 teaspoons red chili powder
- 2 teaspoons paprika
- 1½ teaspoons salt, or to taste
- 1½ teaspoons onion powder
- 1 teaspoon cumin

- ½ teaspoon cayenne pepper
- ½ teaspoon garlic powder
- ½ teaspoon white sugar
- ¼ teaspoon oregano, ground

Directions

1. Mix all the spices in a bowl and store in a glass jar.

Nutrition 1 Calories 0.3g total fat 0.5g Protein

Mrs. Dash Salt-Free Seasoning Mix

Preparation Time: 5 minutes

Cooking Time: 0 minute

Servings: 2

Ingredients

- 2 teaspoons onion powder
- 2 teaspoons black pepper
- 2 teaspoons parsley
- 2 teaspoons dry celery seed
- 1 teaspoon dry basil
- 1 teaspoon dry bay leaf
- 2 teaspoons marjoram
- 2 teaspoons oregano
- 2 teaspoons savory
- 2 teaspoons thyme
- 2 teaspoons cayenne pepper
- 1 teaspoon coriander
- 2 teaspoons cumin
- 1 teaspoon mustard powder
- 2 teaspoons rosemary
- 2 teaspoons garlic powder
- 1 teaspoon mace

Directions

1. Mix all the spices in a bowl and store in a glass jar. Keep it dry.

Nutrition 23 Calories 0.8g total fat 4g carbohydrates0.9g Protein

Old Bay Seasoning

Preparation Time: 4 minutes

Cooking Time: 0 minute

Servings: 4

Ingredients

- ¼ cup bay leaf powder
- ¼ cup celery salt
- 2 tablespoons dry mustard
- 4 teaspoons black pepper, ground
- 4 teaspoons ginger, ground
- 4 teaspoons paprika, smoked
- 2 teaspoons white pepper, ground
- 2 Teaspoons nutmeg, ground
- 2 teaspoons cloves, ground
- 2 teaspoons allspice, ground
- 1 teaspoon crushed red pepper flakes
- 1 teaspoon mace, ground
- 1 teaspoon cardamom, ground
- ½ teaspoon cinnamon, ground

Directions

1. Mix all the spices in a bowl and store in a glass jar. Keep it dry.

Nutrition 16 Calories0.7g total fat 0.6g Protein

DESSERT RECIPES

Pumpkin Cheesecake

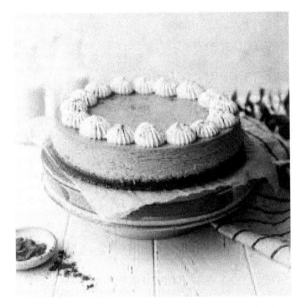

Preparation Time: 8 hours

Cooking Time: 1 hour and 45 minutes

Servings: 8 - 10

Ingredients

- 2 ½ cups graham cracker crumbs
- ¾ cup unsalted butter, melted
- 2 ¾ cups granulated sugar, divided

- 1 teaspoon salt, plus a pinch
- 4 (8-oz) blocks cream cheese, at room temp
- ¼ cup sour cream
- 1 (15-oz) can pure pumpkin
- 6 large eggs, room temperature
- 1 tablespoon vanilla extract
- 2 ½ teaspoons ground cinnamon
- 1 teaspoon ginger, ground
- ¼ teaspoon cloves, ground
- 2 cups whipped cream, sweetened
- 1/3 cup toasted pecans, roughly chopped

Direction

1. Prep the oven to 325°F and grease a 12-inch spring form pan.
2. In a mixing bowl, combine the graham cracker crumbs, melted butter, ¼ cup of the sugar, and a pinch of salt. Mix until well combined and press the mixture into the prepared spring form pan. Bake for about 25 minutes.
3. While baking, scourge cream cheese, sour cream, and pumpkin.
4. Add the rest of the sugar, and slowly incorporate the beaten eggs and vanilla. Add the remaining salt, cinnamon, ginger, and cloves.

5. Fill a large baking pan (big enough to hold your springform pan) with about half an inch of water. Situate it in the oven and let the water get hot.

6. Put foil around the edges of your springform pan, then add the filling and place the pan in the oven with the water bath you made.

7. Bake for 1 hour and 45 minutes, or until the center is set. You can turn the foil over the edges of the cake if it starts to get too brown. Pull out pan from the oven and place it on a cooling rack for one hour before taking out the sides of the springform pan.

8. After it has cooled, remove sides of the pan and refrigerate the cheesecake for at least 8 hours or overnight. Serve with whipped cream and toasted pecans.

Nutrition: 45g Carbohydrates 12g fats 5g protein

Reese's Peanut Butter Chocolate Cake Cheesecake

Preparation Time: 6 hours

Cooking Time: 1 hour 15 minutes

Servings: 8 - 10

Ingredients

Cheesecake

- 4 (8-ounce) packages cream cheese, softened
- 1 ¼ cups sugar
- ½ cup sour cream
- 2 teaspoons vanilla extract
- 5 eggs
- 8 Chocolate Peanut Butter cups, chopped
- 1 (14-ounce) can dulce de leche

Chocolate Cake

- 1 ¾ cups all-purpose flour
- 2 cups sugar
- ¾ cup cocoa
- 2 teaspoons baking soda
- 1 teaspoon salt
- 2 eggs, room temp
- 1 cup buttermilk
- ½ cup butter, melted

- 1 tablespoon vanilla extract
- 1 cup black coffee, hot

Peanut Butter Buttercream

- ¾ cup butter
- ¾ cup shortening
- ¾ cup peanut butter
- 1 ½ teaspoons vanilla
- 4-5 cups powdered sugar

Ganache

- 2 cups semi-sweet chocolate chips
- 1 cup heavy cream
- 1 teaspoon vanilla

Directions

1. Prep the oven to 350°F and brush 9-inch springform pan. Make the cheesecake. Preheat the oven to 475°F. Fill a large baking pan (your springform pan with have to fit in it) with half an inch of water and place it in the oven while it preheats.

2. Beat the cream cheese in a large bowl until it is fluffy. Gradually incorporate the sugar, sour cream, and vanilla, and mix well.

3. Scourge eggs one at a time and beat until just combined. Fold in the peanut butter cups and pour the batter into the springform pan. Bake at

475°F for 15 minutes, and reduce the heat to 350°F and bake for 60 minutes.

4. Pull out the cake from the oven and cool for 60 minutes before taking off the sides of the springform pan. When it is completely cool, refrigerate the cheesecake for at least 6 hours, but 8 hours to overnight would be better. When it is completely cold, cut the cheesecake in half to make two layers.

5. Meanwhile, make the chocolate cake: mix the flour, sugar, cocoa, baking soda, and salt together in a large bowl. Mix in the eggs, buttermilk, melted butter, and vanilla, and beat until it is smooth. Slowly incorporate the coffee.

6. Coat and flour two 9-inch round cake pans. Pour the batter evenly into each pan and bake for 30–35 minutes. When fully cooked, remove the cakes from the oven and cool for 15 minutes before taking them out of the pans. When fully cooled, wrap each cake in plastic wrap and refrigerate until ready to assemble the cake.

7. Scourge butter and shortening, then add the peanut butter and vanilla. Sprinkle powdered sugar one cup at a time until you achieve the desired sweetness and consistency.

8. To assemble, put one layer of chocolate cake on a cake plate. Drizzle half of the dulce de leche over the top of the cake. Top that with a layer of cheesecake, and spread peanut butter frosting over the top of the cheesecake. Repeat to make a second layer. When assembled, place the whole cake in the freezer for about an hour to fully set.

9. Make the ganache by melting chocolate chips with heavy cream and vanilla in a small saucepan. When the cake is completely set, pour ganache over the top. Refrigerate until ganache the sets.

Nutrition: 42g Carbohydrates 13g fats 5g protein

White Chocolate Raspberry Swirl Cheesecake

Preparation Time: 5 hours

Cooking Time: 1 hour 15 minutes

Servings: 8 - 10

Ingredients

Crust

- 1 ½ cups chocolate cookie crumbs, such as crumbled Oreo® cookies
- 1/3 cup butter, melted

Filling

- 4 (8-ounce) packages cream cheese
- 1 ¼ cups granulated sugar
- ½ cup sour cream
- 2 teaspoons vanilla extract
- ½ cup raspberry preserves (or raspberry pie filling)
- ¼ cup water
- 5 eggs
- 4 ounces white chocolate, chopped into chunks

Optional Garnish

- 2 ounces shaved white chocolate (optional)
- Fresh whipped cream

Directions

1. Preheat the oven to 475°F. In a food processor, crumble the cookies and add the melted butter. Press the mixture into a greased 9-inch springform pan, and place in the freezer while you make the filling.

2. Stir in half an inch of water in a large baking pan and situate it in the oven. Scourge together the cream cheese, sugar, sour cream, and vanilla. Scrape the sides of the bowl after the ingredients have been well combined.

3. Whisk eggs in a small bowl then add them slowly to the cream cheese mixture.

4. In another small dish, mix the raspberry preserves and water. Microwave for 1 minute.

5. Pull out the crust from the freezer then cover the outside bottom of the pan with aluminum foil. Sprinkle the white chocolate over the crust, then pour half of the cheesecake batter into the springform pan. Next, drizzle half of the raspberry preserves over the top of the batter. Then add the rest of the batter with the rest of the drizzle.

6. Situate springform pan into the water bath and bake for 15 minutes at 475°F, then decrease the

heat to 350°F then bake for 60 more minutes more

7. Remove from oven and cool it completely before removing sides of pan, then move to the refrigerator for at least 5 hours. Serve with extra white chocolate and fresh whipped cream.

Nutrition: 41g Carbohydrates 12g fats 4g protein

Carrot Cake Cheesecake

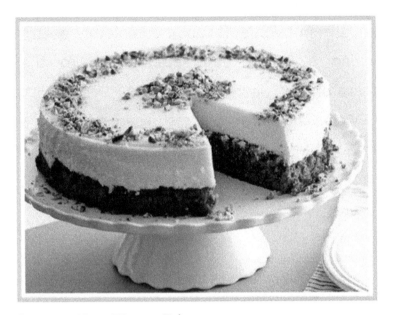

Preparation Time: 5 hours

Cooking Time: 58 minutes

Servings: 8

Ingredients

Cheesecake

- 2 (8-oz) blocks cream cheese, at room temp
- ¾ cup granulated sugar
- 1 tablespoon flour
- 3 eggs
- 1 teaspoon vanilla

Carrot Cake

- ¾ cup vegetable oil
- 1 cup granulated sugar

- 2 eggs
- 1 teaspoon vanilla
- 1 cup flour
- 1 teaspoon baking soda
- 1 teaspoon cinnamon
- 1 dash salt
- 1 (8-oz) can crushed pineapple
- 1 cup grated carrot
- ½ cup flaked coconut
- ½ cup chopped walnuts

Pineapple Cream Cheese Frosting

- 2 ounces cream cheese, softened
- 1 tablespoon butter, softened
- 1 ¾ cups powdered sugar
- ½ teaspoon vanilla
- 1 tablespoon reserved pineapple juice

Directions

1. Prep the oven to 350°F and coat a 9-inch springform pan. Scourge cream cheese and the sugar until smooth. Incorporate flour, eggs, and vanilla until well combined. Set aside.

2. In another large bowl, beat together the ¾ cup vegetable oil, sugar, eggs and vanilla until smooth. Then add the flour, baking soda, cinnamon and salt and beat until smooth. Fold in

the crushed pineapple, grated carrot, coconut, and walnuts.

3. Pour 1 ½ cups of the carrot cake batter into the prepared pan. Drop large spoonful of the cream cheese batter over the top of the carrot cake batter. Then add spoonful of carrot cake batter over the top of the cream cheese batter. Repeat with the remaining batter.

4. Bake the cake for 58 minutes. Take it from the oven and cool for about an hour before taking the sides off the springform pan. Refrigerate for at least 5 hours.

5. Beating together all the frosting ingredients. Garnish the cake when it is completely cool.

Nutrition: 40g Carbohydrates 11g fats 6g protein

Original Cheesecake

Preparation Time: 4 hours 15 minutes

Cooking Time: 1 hour 5 minutes

Servings: 12

Ingredients

Crust:

- 1 ½ cups graham cracker crumbs
- ¼ teaspoon ground cinnamon
- 1/3 cup margarine, melted

Filling:

- 4 (8-ounce) packages cream cheese, softened
- 1 ¼ cups white sugar
- ½ cup sour cream
- 2 teaspoons vanilla extract
- 5 large eggs

Topping:

- ½ cup sour cream
- 2 teaspoons sugar

Directions:

1. Set the oven to 475°F then situate a skillet with half an inch of water inside. Incorporate ingredients for the crust in a bowl. Line a large pie pan with parchment paper, and spread crust

onto pan. Press firmly. Wrap with foil, and keep it in the freezer until ready to use.

2. Combine all the ingredients for the filling EXCEPT the eggs in a bowl. Scoop the sides of the bowl while beating, until mixture is smooth. Mix in eggs one at a time, and beat until fully blended.

3. Take the crust from the freezer then pour in the filling, spreading it evenly. Place the pie pan into the heated skillet in the oven, and bake for about 12 minutes.

4. Reduce the heat to 350°F. Continue to bake for about 50 minutes, or until the top of the cake is golden. Pull away from the oven and transfer the skillet onto a wire rack to cool.

5. Prepare the topping by mixing all ingredients in a bowl. Coat the cake with the topping, then cover. Refrigerate for at least 4 hours. Serve cold.

Nutrition: 41g Carbohydrates 11g fats 2g protein

Ultimate Red Velvet Cheesecake

Preparation Time: 3 hours 30 minutes

Cooking Time: 1 hour 15 minutes

Servings: 16

Ingredients

Cheesecake:

- 2 (8-ounce) packages cream cheese, softened
- 2/3 cup granulated white sugar
- Pinch salt
- 2 large eggs
- 1/3 cup sour cream
- 1/3 cup heavy whipping cream
- 1 teaspoon vanilla extract
- Non-stick cooking spray
- Hot water, for water bath

Red velvet cake:

- 2 ½ cups all-purpose flour
- 1 ½ cups granulated white sugar
- 3 tablespoons unsweetened cocoa powder
- 1 ½ teaspoons baking soda
- 1 teaspoon salt
- 2 large eggs
- 1 ½ cups vegetable oil
- 1 cup buttermilk

- ¼ cup red food coloring
- 2 teaspoons vanilla extract
- 2 teaspoons white vinegar

Frosting:
- 2 ½ cups powdered sugar, sifted
- 2 (8-ounce) packages cream cheese, softened
- ½ cup unsalted butter, softened
- 1 tablespoon vanilla extract

Directions:

1. For the cheesecake, set the oven to 325°F. Beat the cream cheese, sugar, and salt for about 2 minutes, until creamy and smooth. Add the eggs, mixing again after adding each one. Add the sour cream, heavy cream, and vanilla extract, and beat until smooth and well blended.

2. Brush springform pan with non-stick cooking spray, then place parchment paper on top. Wrap the outsides entirely with two layers of aluminum foil.

3. Pour the cream cheese batter into the pan, then place it in a roasting pan. Fill in boiling water to the roasting pan to surround the springform pan. Situate it in the oven and bake for 45 minutes, until set.

4. Transfer the springform pan with the cheesecake onto a rack to cool for about 1 hour. Refrigerate overnight.

5. For the red velvet cake, prep the oven to 350°F. Combine the flour, sugar, cocoa powder, baking soda, and salt in a large bowl. Scourge eggs, oil, buttermilk, food coloring, vanilla and vinegar. Add the wet ingredients to dry ingredients. Blend for 1 minute with a mixer on medium-low speed, then on high speed for 2 minutes.

6. Spray non-stick cooking spray in 2 metal baking pans that are the same size as the springform pan used for the cheesecake. Coat the bottoms thinly with flour. Divide the batter between them.

7. Bake for about 30–35 minutes. The cake is done when only a few crumbs attach to a toothpick when inserted in the center. Situate the cakes to a rack and let them cool for 10 minutes. Separate the cakes from the pans using a knife around the edges, then invert them onto the rack. Let them cool completely.

8. To prepare the frosting, mix the powdered sugar, cream cheese, butter, and vanilla using a mixer on medium-high speed, just until smooth.

9. Assemble the cake by positioning one red velvet cake layer onto a cake plate. Take out the cheesecake from the pan, peel off the parchment paper, and layer it on top of the red velvet cake layer. Top with the second red velvet cake layer.

10. Coat a thin layer of prepared frosting on the entire outside of the cake. Clean the spatula every time you scoop out from bowl of frosting, so as to not mix crumbs into it. Refrigerate for 30 minutes to set. Then coat cake the with a second layer by adding a large scoop on top then spreading it to the top side of the cake then around it. Cut into slices. Serve.

Nutrition: 39g Carbohydrates 12g fats 4g protein

Strawberry Shortcake

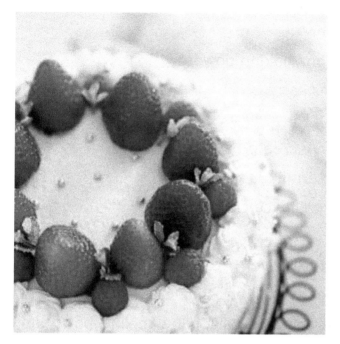

Preparation Time: 5 minutes

Cooking Time: 2 hours and 15 minutes

Servings: 16

Ingredients

Sugared Strawberries:

- 2 cups strawberries (sliced)
- ¼ cup granulated sugar

Whipped Cream:

- 4 cups heavy cream
- ½ cup powdered sugar
- ¼ teaspoon vanilla

Shortcake Biscuit:

- 4 ½ cups all-purpose flour
- ½ cup sugar
- 5 tablespoons baking powder
- 2 teaspoons salt
- 1 ¾ cups butter
- 2 cups heavy cream
- 2 cups buttermilk
- 2 scoops vanilla ice cream

Directions

1. Preheat the oven to 375°F. Mix sliced strawberries with the sugar. Stir, cover, and refrigerate for 2 hours. Chill a mixing bowl and beat the heavy cream, powdered sugar, and vanilla until soft peaks form. Refrigerate.

2. Scourge flour, sugar, baking powder, and salt. Stir to combine. With two butter knives, cut the butter into the flour mixture until it becomes crumbly. Add the cream and the buttermilk and mix gently until the batter forms.

3. Spread out the dough onto a prep surface to form biscuits about half an inch thick. Take care not to turn the cutter as you remove it from the dough. Place the biscuits on a non-stick cookie

sheet and bake for about 15 minutes. They should at least double in size.

4. When they cool, assemble the shortcake by cutting each biscuit in half, topping the bottom half with strawberries and ice cream, and placing the top half of the biscuit on top of the ice cream. Top with more strawberries and whipped cream.

Nutrition: 40g Carbohydrates 12g fats 5g protein

Limoncello Cream Torte

Preparation Time: 15 minutes

Cooking Time: 20 minutes plus 5 hours chilling time

Servings: 8 - 10

Ingredients

- 1 box yellow cake mix
- Limoncello liqueur (optional)
- 1 package ladyfinger cookies
- 1 (3-ounce) package sugar-free lemon gelatin
- 1 cup boiling water
- 1 (8-ounce) package cream cheese, softened
- 1 teaspoon vanilla extract
- 1 (13-ounce) can cold milnot (evaporated milk), whipped

For the glaze:

- 1 cup confectioner's sugar
- 1–2 tablespoons lemon juice

Directions

1. Preheat the oven to 350°F. Prep the yellow cake mix following to the directions on the package. Use two 9-inch round cake pans, or you can use a springform pan and cut the cake in half after it is baked.

---

2. Once cooled, you can soak the layers lightly with some limoncello. Do the same with the ladyfingers. Fill in 1 cup of water then stir in the lemon gelatin. Refrigerate until it gets thick, but don't let it set.

3. Mix together the cream cheese and vanilla, then mix in the thickened gelatin. Fold the whipped milnot into the mixture until combined. To assemble the cake, place the bottom layer of the cake back in the pan. This will help you get even layers. Top the cake with about half an inch of the lemon filling. Place ladyfingers on top of the filling, then top with another layer of the filling. Situate the other half of the cake on the top.

4. Place the cake in the refrigerator to set. Make a drizzle with some lemon juice and confectioner's sugar, and drizzle over the cake.

Nutrition: 45g Carbohydrates 16g fats 5g protein

Oreo Cookie Cheesecake

Preparation Time: 6 hours

Cooking Time: 60 minutes

Servings: 8 - 10

Ingredients

- 1 package Oreo cookies
- 1/3 cup unsalted butter, melted
- 3 (8-ounce) packages cream cheese
- ¾ cup granulated sugar
- 4 eggs
- 1 cup sour cream
- 1 teaspoon vanilla extract
- Whipped cream and additional cookies for garnish

Directions

1. Preheat the oven to 350°F. Crush most of the cookies (25-30) in a food processor or blender, and add the melted butter. Push down cookie mixture into the bottom of a 9-inch springform pan and keep it in the refrigerator while you prepare the filling.
2. Scourge cream cheese until smooth, and add the sugar. Beat in the eggs in one a time. When

the eggs are mixed together, beat in the sour cream and vanilla.

3. Chop the remaining cookies and fold them gently into the filling mixture. Transfer filling into the springform pan and bake at 350°F for 50–60 minutes. Ensure the center of the cake has set.

4. Let the cake cool for 15 minutes, then carefully remove the sides of the springform pan. Transfer to the refrigerator and refrigerate for 4–6 hours or overnight.

Nutrition: 47g Carbohydrates 18g fats 8g protein

BEVERAGE RECIPES

Olive Garden Green Apple Moscato Sangria

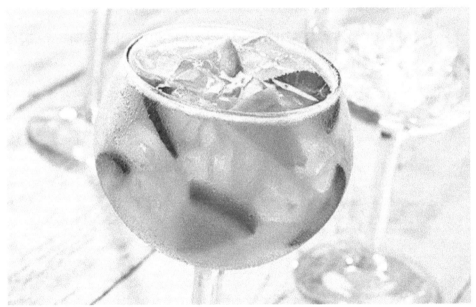

Preparation Time: 11 minutes

Cooking Time: 0 minutes

Servings: 6

Ingredients

- 750 ml Moscato
- Puree or Apple Pucker

- 8 cups ice
- 1/2 cup strawberries
- 1/2 cup orange slices
- 1/2 cup green apple slices

Direction

1. In a large pitcher combine chilled Moscato, pineapple juice, and granny smith apple puree. Stir until well combined 6 ounces pineapple juice
2. Serve by placing several ice cubes in a glass, pour beverage 6 ounces Granny Smith Apple over ice.

Nutrition: 59 Calories 0.5g Protein 0.21g Fat

Olive Garden Sangria

Preparation Time: 9 minutes

Cooking Time: 0 minutes

Servings: 10

Ingredients

- Liters Red Table Wine
- 12 ounces sweet vermouth
- 10 ounces simple syrup (5 ounces sugar diluted in 5 ounces water)

Direction

1. Mix all ingredients except for ice. Pour sangria in glass and then add ice. Make sure there is fruit in every glass.

Nutrition: 195 Calories 0.85g Protein 0.28g Fat

Refreshing Olive Garden Peach Iced Tea

Preparation Time: 11 minutes

Cooking Time: 0 minutes

Servings: 6

Ingredients

For Peach Syrup

- 2-4 fresh peaches, pitted and sliced
- 1 C. sugar
- 1 C. water

For Tea

- 5½ C. boiling water
- 2-3 tea bags

Directions

2. For peach syrup: in a pan add all ingredients over medium-high heat and bring to a boil.
3. Reduce the heat to medium and cook until sugar is dissolved, crushing the peach slices occasionally.
4. Remove from heat and keep aside, covered for about 30 minutes.
5. Through a strainer, strain the syrup and discard the solids.

6. For brewing tea: in a pan of boiling water, steep the tea bags for about 5-6 minutes.

7. Remove the tea bags and keep aside to cool completely before using.

8. Add peach syrup and stir to combine.

9. Serve the tea over ice.

Nutrition: 90 Calories 0.53g Protein 0.6g Fat

Watermelon Moscato Sangria

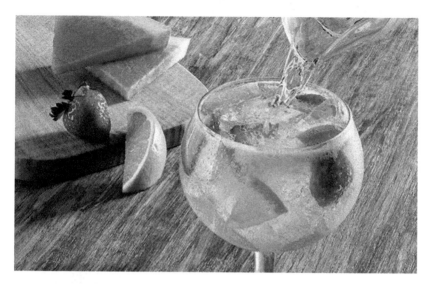

Preparation Time: 12 minutes

Cooking Time: 0 minutes

Servings: 6

Ingredients

- 750 ml Moscato
- 6 ounces Ginger Ale
- 6 ounces Monin Watermelon
- 4 cups ice
- 3/4 cup sliced strawberries
- 1 orange sliced

Direction

1. Wash and cut fruit into small slices.
2. Pour Moscato into a large pitcher.

3. Pour Ginger Ale and Watermelon syrup into a pitcher. Stir Syrup gently.
4. Add ice to the pitcher, and stir gently.
5. Add sliced strawberries and oranges.
6. Serve with watermelon slices if desired.

Nutrition: 37 Calories 0.8g Protein 0.3g Fat

Tropical Margarita

Preparation Time: 10 minutes

Cooking Time: 10 minutes

Servings: 2

Ingredients

- 1 ½ cups mango chunks, frozen
- ¼ cup liquid (pineapple juice, coconut water or orange juice)
- 1 tablespoon orange liqueur
- 2 tablespoons lime juice, freshly squeezed
- ¼ cup coconut, shredded or finely chopped
- 1 cup pineapple chunks, frozen
- ½ cup silver tequila
- Lime wedges

Directions

1. Add mango chunks with pineapple chunks to a blender.
2. Pour in the orange liqueur, tequila, and lime juice.
3. Blend on high until smooth, for a minute or two. Slowly add in the liquid until you have a smooth cocktail.
4. Dip or rub the rim of 2 margarita glasses with the freshly squeezed lime juice.

5. Dip the glass rim into the coconut shreds.

6. Now, fill the glasses with the margarita and garnish each glass with lime wedges.

Nutrition: 39 Calories 0.4g Protein 0.1g Fat

Milan Mai Tai

Preparation Time: 5 minutes

Cooking Time: 5 minutes

Servings: 1

Ingredients

- 1 teaspoon grenadine syrup
- ½ jigger coconut-flavored rum (1.5 fluid ounce)
- 3 fluid ounces pineapple juice
- 1 jigger spiced rum (1.5 fluid ounce)
- 2 fluid ounces orange juice
- 1 cup ice cubes

Directions

1. Fill a cocktail mixer with ice cubes and then combine the coconut rum with spiced rum, grenadine, orange juice and pineapple juice. Shake vigorously & strain into the glass full of ice cubes.

Nutrition: 47 Calories 4g Protein 2g Fat

Peach Bellini

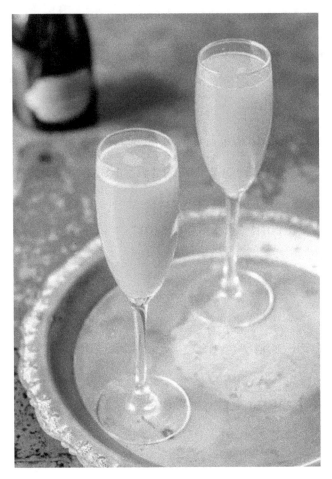

Preparation Time: 10 minutes

Cooking Time: 10 minutes

Servings: 6

Ingredients

- 1 tablespoon lemon juice, freshly squeezed
- 2 peaches, ripe, seeded & diced
- 1 bottle prosecco sparkling wine, chilled

- 1 teaspoon sugar

Directions

1. Place peaches with sugar and lemon juice in the food processor bowl fitted with a steel blade; process on high until smooth, for a minute or two.
2. Press the mixture through a sieve; discarding the peach solids in the sieve. Place 2 tablespoons of peach puree into each Champagne glass & fill with cold prosecco.
3. Serve immediately & enjoy.

Nutrition: 32 Calories 1g Protein 0.2g Fat

Peach Sangria

Preparation Time: 5 minutes

Cooking Time: 2 hours & 10 minutes

Servings: 6

Ingredients

- 6 tablespoons lemonade concentrate, frozen & thawed
- ¾ cup peach flavored vodka
- 1 bottle dry white wine (750 milliliter)
- ¾ cup each red and green grape, seedless & halved
- 1-pound white peaches, pitted & sliced
- ¼ cup white sugar

Directions

1. Combine dry white wine with lemonade concentrate, peach vodka and sugar in a large pitcher. Stir until sugar is completely dissolved and then add in the sliced peaches, green and red grapes.

2. Refrigerate the sangria for a minimum period of 2 hours, until well chilled. For best flavors, you can refrigerate the sangria for overnight. Serve over ice and don't forget to include some sliced

---

peaches & grapes with every serving using a
slotted spoon.

Nutrition: 28 Calories 7g Protein 2g Fat

Moscato Citrus Berry Cocktail

Preparation Time: 5 minutes

Cooking Time: 5 minutes

Servings: 2

Ingredients

- 20 blueberries, fresh & smashed
- Barefoot Moscato Spumante
- Lemon wedges & Blueberries for garnish
- Juice of ½ lemon, freshly squeezed

Directions

1. Pour freshly squeezed lemon juice in a large glass.
2. Using a fine strainer; mash the blueberries and release its juices, then add the juice to the glass.
3. Fill the glass with ice cubes approximately ¾ full.
4. Pour in the Moscato & garnish with lemon wedge and some of the blueberries.

Nutrition: 47 Calories 9g Protein 3g Fat

CONCLUSION

Creativity often happens when you cook at home, and you can attach a range of plant foods to a variety of colors. The copycat recipes are perfect for the dishes you want to recreate.

But, watch out. Everyone has their favorite dishes, and others love to have a bite of their world-famous recipes. Will you be the first to make a copycat recipe that tastes the same as the original recipe? Or will you mix in the wrong ingredients, and damage the recipe so that you end up with a concoction that tastes weird?

You need to have all your ingredients collection, mix them up and see how you can make the taste just like the original recipe.

Serving control from home can be regulated. Once the food is cooked for us, we tend to eat all or most of it.

Try to use little dishes at home, but ensure that all good things like vegetables, fruits, whole grains, and legumes are filled. You are certainly going to be satisfied and happy.

The major advantage of trying copycat restaurant recipes is that you can save more money and use your creativity to improve the dish. You can also adjust the ingredients and add those favorite herbs to your desired taste. Now you have saved your money and restaurant-quality dishes for your family as well.

You may not include some ingredients of your favorite dish when you try the copycat recipes, and it is okay. Following the recipe while recreating your favorite dish is what we are here for.

It is not hard to acquire those top-secret restaurant-quality recipes. Others may advise that you need to have culinary credentials to cook those secret recipes. Yet, we can gather those ingredients ourselves and cook an elaborate meal that tastes like the real deal.

But do top secret restaurant recipes taste the way the chef served them? Perhaps. You can easily recreate your favorite recipes with patience and a little practice.

You may start to think that some recipes need additional seasonings to improve your dish than the original. Nevertheless, if you wanted to prepare this dish on your own, there is still a chance.

Just a few simple tips and tricks, you can also make quality cuisine in your kitchen. These tricks may not seem so strong on their own but can transform how you prepare and produce food when they are all used together. These tips help you cook at home like a pro from expired spices and how you use salt to arrange it before you start cooking.

When preparing desserts at home, you can tweak the recipes as you wish. As you sample the recipes, you will know the usual ingredients and techniques in making popular sweet treats.

It could inspire you to create your very own recipes. You can use alternative ingredients according to your taste, budget or health.

You can come up, possibly, not with a dish that is perfectly alike as the restaurant's recipe, but with one that is exactly the way you want it to be.

Most of all, the recipes here are meant for you to experience the contentment of seeing those smiles on the people whom you share with your dishes or creations. Keep cooking and have fun with the recipes, and soon, you will be reaping your sweet rewards!

If prepared food reaches outside the home, you typically have limited knowledge about salt, sugar, and processed oils. For a fact, we also apply more to our meal when it is served to the table. You will say how much salt, sugar, and oil are being used to prepare meals at home.

Copycat recipes practically give you the ability to make great restaurant food tasting in your own home and get it the right first time and easily.

Lightning Source UK Ltd.
Milton Keynes UK
UKHW021821160421
382091UK00005B/86